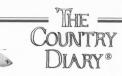

THE COUNTRY DIARY®

Herbal Remedies

Written by David Holzer

Illustrations by Edith Holden,
Gail Glaser, Liz Hankins, and Sally Pinhey

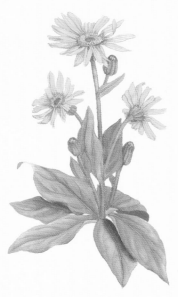

TOP THAT!

First published in the United States and Canada in 2006 by Top That! Publishing Inc,

25031 W. Avenue Stanford, Suite 60, Valencia, CA 91355.

www.topthatpublishing.com

0 2 4 6 8 9 7 5 3 1

ISBN 1-84666-021-1

Color reproduction by Reflex Reproduction

Printed and bound in China

Acknowledgments and Credits:

Managing Director Barrie Henderson

Kudos Manager Mike Saiz

Designer David Freeland

Senior Editor Karen Rigden

Junior Editor Duncan Ballantyne-Way

Photography Jo Broome and Top Foto (p 21)

Illustrations: Gail Glaser p 26 and p 32, Liz Hankins p 45, p 46, and p 47,

Sally Pinhey p 1, p 36, p 42, and p 44. All other illustrations by Edith Holden.

Contents

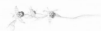

A Note from the Publisher

The remedies featured in this book are based on traditional recipes. While they have been used by generations of people, not all of their benefits have been proven scientifically, as such the publisher cannot guarantee the effectiveness of the remedies featured herein. As a precaution, the publisher strongly recommends that you use the remedies with care—following the advice when given—and performing a patch test (see page 6) before applying any remedies directly to the skin. If in doubt of your own sensitivity to an ingredient please consult a doctor or trained herbalist before proceeding. If you suffer from epilepsy, are pregnant, or breast-feeding it is recommended that you seek professional advice before using these remedies. Self-diagnosis and treatment should only be used for the most minor of ailments, those suffering from serious or long-term illnesses or conditions should consult a doctor. The use of herbal remedies should be avoided while taking any course of prescribed medication unless advised otherwise by a professional. If any adverse reactions occur seek medical advice immediately.

Introducing
Herbal Remedies

For centuries herbs have been used to treat the body and mind to keep both healthy. Today, millions of people are choosing to use medicines and preparations made with herbs as a natural alternative to conventional medicines.

Botanically speaking, a herb is a seed plant that does not produce a woody stem like a tree, but lives long enough to develop flowers and seeds. It's very easy to find prepared herbal remedies in specialist stores and supermarkets. However, growing your own herbs and making your own remedies, is great fun and a lot more satisfying. It's also an excellent way to find out about the natural world.

During the Edwardian era these herbal remedies would have already been passed on from generation to generation by word of mouth. This book brings to you some of the most recognized and useful recipes in an easy-to-follow and clear manner, using beautiful watercolor illustrations by Edith Holden.

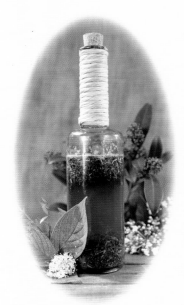

The identification of herbs is a trained skill in itself. Historically, trial and error were used to discover the medicinal properties of herbs, how much to use and which part of the herb was safe. However, today the safest way to use herbs is to buy them from a trained herbalist or to grow your own, ensuring that the plant or seed is bought from a reputable source who will have correctly identified them. If in any doubt as to the identity of a herb do not use it.

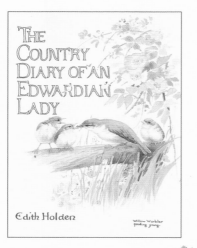

The Country Diary

Herbal Remedies has been inspired by the elegance and beauty of *The Country Diary of an Edwardian Lady*®, whose author, Edith Holden, was born in 1871. In her lifetime she was an artist and art teacher. She was also very well known for her illustrations for children's books. Although *The Country Diary of an Edwardian Lady*® was published 1977, it is actually a naturalist's diary for the year 1906. In the course of that year, Edith recorded the seasonal changes of the British countryside in words and delicate, delightful watercolors.

When it was found and published in 1977, readers were captivated by its charm and evocation of a simpler world. It has now been translated into 13 different languages and has sold millions of copies worldwide.

Tragically, Edith was to die in 1920, at the age of 49. Collecting flowers from a riverbank at Kew Gardens in Richmond near London, she fell into the River Thames and drowned.

Buying Herbs and Remedies

With the growing popularity of alternative health remedies buying prepared ingredients has never been easier. The safest place to buy your herbs, in particular dried ones, but also prepared tinctures, capsules, and ointments, is from any of the well-known main street health stores. Independent, new-age shops are also a good place to look and the assistants may be able to offer you additional advice and information. The internet is another option, but buy and use the purchased products with due caution. With any product read the label carefully before use, following any of the listed precautions and, in particular, note the concentration of the remedy and use accordingly.

Skin Safety

As with any cosmetic or medicine, some people may react adversely to remedies that are applied directly to the skin. It is therefore strongly advisable that you test your skin for sensitivity to any new remedy with a patch test first.

Patch Test

Apply a small amount of the remedy to the inside of your wrist and leave for 24 hours. If there are no visible signs of irritation, or if you do not experience any discomfort, the remedy is safe to use. If you do have an adverse reaction discontinue use immediately and seek medical advice.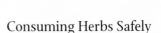

Consuming Herbs Safely

Teas and remedies that are ingested should be used with caution as well. If you experience food allergies seek advice or use a weaker concoction of the remedy first.

As with an allergic reaction of the skin, if you experience any discomfort after consuming a remedy discontinue use immediately and seek medical advice.

Using Herbs

Different remedies and methods of preparation require different parts of the herb. You may need to use the whole of the plant or just the root, leaves, flowers, or fruit.

Using Roots, Leaves, and Blossoms

The root of a herb is usually ground to a powder unless you're making a tincture, decoction, or syrup, when the root needs to be cut up into small chunks. If the leaf is required you will either need to use the whole leaf or, if you're preparing a tea, you'll have to crumple it first. The same is true for flowers and blossoms. Many of the plants featured in this book are actually available in the retail market; in raw or dried form, as well as in manufactured products (tinctures, extracts, capsules, etc.) —the quality of these products does, however, vary enormously so shop wisely.

Correctly Identifying Herbs

Most herbs are now classified as wild plants and should never be picked from the countryside. This provides a useful safety net to stop people identifying the herb incorrectly and accidentally poisoning themselves. There are many poisonous plants that look like the beneficial herb, so always leave them well alone. Growing your own herbs from seed is a safe way to ensure you use the right herb. Mistakes are made, however, and you can never be entirely sure unless you buy them from a trained herbalist or an established commercial store.

Herbal Remedies and Medicines

Many herbs—chamomile, for instance—are not particularly powerful, certainly in small doses. However some, such as St John's wort, are rather more potent and can interact badly with conventional drugs; so if in doubt, consult a doctor or herbalist first.

Growing, Gathering, and Drying Herbs

Growing, gathering, and drying herbs yourself ensures that they are always fresh and have been properly prepared.

Creating an Outdoor Herb Garden

A herb garden requires well-draining soil as herbs won't grow in wet soil. It is also a good idea to avoid especially fertile soil which can produce lush, dense herbs but with only the mildest of flavor.

Sowing Herb Seed

You can grow nearly all herbs from seeds. Sow your seeds in shallow boxes in late winter and plant the seedlings outside in spring—about an inch below the surface.

Growing Herbs Indoors

It's no more difficult to grow herbs indoors than out. You just need sunlight and thoroughly drained, not too rich, soil. Place your herbs near a south or west-facing window and, in winter, use a fluorescent light or grow lamp. Plant them in a mixture of two parts sterilized potting soil and one part sand. For good drainage, lay down a base of gravel. Ensure your herbs have enough water without drenching them.

When to Harvest

It's always best to harvest mid-morning. Picking leaves or seeds after the dew has disappeared but before the sun is too hot guarantees a fair amount of oil (in which the main medicinal properties are found). When harvesting leaves to dry them, harvest before the flower buds open. Seed heads should be picked as the color changes from green to brown. Roots and bark should be gathered in early spring when the plant is beginning to show leaf buds, or in fall when the leaves are turning.

Drying Herbs

All herbs must be dried thoroughly if you want to store them for any length of time. Before drying, remember to wash your herbs in cold running water, drain them and leave them to air-dry on newspaper or paper towels.

To then fully dry them, find a dark, warm, well-ventilated, and dust-free area. If you're only drying the leaves, strip all but the top 6 inches from a plant, take off all blossoms and hang a sizeable bunch of the plant upside down in a brown paper bag. You'll know the leaves are ready when they feel dry and crumbly—usually after about one to two weeks.

Seeds take longer to dry than leaves. Dry them by hanging the whole plant upside down inside a brown paper bag, this catches the seeds as they dry and fall off.

You can also dry herbs using your oven. Spread a well-spaced layer on a shallow cookie sheet. The oven should be turned on to its lowest setting—higher temperatures will cook the herbs, if the temperature still seems too hot open the door slightly. Stir the herbs periodically until they are thoroughly dry which can take a few hours depending on the herb.

Storing Dried Herbs

Store your herbs in airtight containers away from light; dark-colored glass jars are ideal. Leaves can be stored whole or reduced to a powder using a pestle and mortar. Seeds should be stored whole and ground as needed.

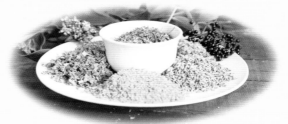

Infusions and Oils

A herbal infusion is made by soaking a herb in boiling water to extract the beneficial properties. The infusion is then drunk like tea. Herbs are also soaked in oil to create infused oils that are then used in other remedies, often to dilute other essential oils before applying them to the skin.

Infusions

Infusions are simple to make and although not all of the medicinal properties of the plant can be extracted with this method, it is a direct and effective way to take a herbal remedy as the body can absorb the tea quickly. There is also the added psychological benefit of drinking a soothing beverage, which can be served hot, warm, cold, or iced.

Although infusions are generally drunk, the process and product of an infusion can also be used in other remedies such as compresses and poultices (pages 16-17).

Whatever the use of the infusion the method is the same, with fresh or dried herbs being steeped in boiling water. This method can be used for flowers, leaves, fine roots and barks, berries, and seeds— suggestions for specific herbs are given later in this book (pages 25, 27, 31, 35, 37, 45, and 47) but for additional herbs ask a trained herbalist.

You will need

- ½-1 tsp dried herbs or 1-2 tsp fresh herbs

- 8 fl oz boiling water

Makes one cup; tea can be drunk up to three times a day, for up to four days.

Method

1. Chop or crush your chosen herb. Pour on the boiling water, then cover and leave to soak for the relevant time according to taste:

• fresh flowers, berries, and leaves: 3-5 mins

• dried or tougher parts: 2-15 mins

2. Strain the mixture, discarding the pulp unless being used for another remedy (for example a poultice), and enjoy the drink.

Infused Oils

While infusions and teas are consumed, infused oils are for external use only and often form part of another remedy such as an ointment, although they can also be massaged into the skin (following a patch test). There are two methods to infuse oils, the cold method is better suited to delicate, aromatic herbs, while the hot method suits tougher herbs. Page 41 features a specific infused oil suggestion. If you wish to try other herbs ask a herbalist for advice.

Cold Method

1. Fill a large jar, with a tight-fitting lid, compactly with herb flowers or leaves.

2. Pour in your infusing vegetable oil until the herbs are covered and screw on the lid. You can use any kind of vegetable oil, such as olive, sesame, or almond.

3. Place the jar on a sunny window sill for 2-4 weeks, shaking the mixture daily.

4. Strain the infused oil through a coffee filter or fine cloth. Repeat the process with fresh herbs for a more potent mixture.

5. Carefully discard any watery residue that collects at the bottom of the mixture before transferring the oil into a dark glass bottle and store in a cool, dark place.

Hot Method

You can use either dried or fresh herbs for this method but you will need twice as much of the fresh herb to oil, for example if you have 8 fl oz of oil you will need 16 fl oz of mashed up herb.

1. Place a glass bowl over a saucepan of simmering water like a bain-marie.

2. Add the herbs and oil (olive, sesame, or almond) and heat over a low setting for 2-3 hours. Strain and replace the herbs after two hours if desired.

3. Strain into a bowl discarding any watery residue. Leave to cool and transfer to dark glass bottles sealed with a cap. Store in a cool, dark place.

Decoctions and Tinctures

Decoctions are used when working with tougher, fibrous herbs. They extract the mineral salts and bitter principles of the herb, rather than the volatile ingredients. Alcoholic tinctures are used when plants have chemicals that are not soluble in water.

Decoction

When your herbal remedy calls for you to use tougher parts of the plant, such as the roots, barks, berries, and stems, you will need to make a decoction. A decoction is an intense way of extracting the active properties of the herb but only using boiling water. Specific remedies can be found on pages 21 and 39, but for other decoctions is it safest to ask a herbalist first.

You will need

• 1½ oz dried or 2 oz fresh herbs

• 2 pints boiling water

Method

1. Chop up the plant material you're using as thinly as possible.

2. Place the herbs in a saucepan with the water and boil the decoction.

3. Simmer the mixture until the volume of liquid has been reduced by about a third, this should take around 20-30 minutes.

4. Strain the mixture.

5. Drink the decoction in a wineglass-sized dose taken three times a day. Store in a sealed jar in a cool, dark place. If you wish, you can reheat the decoction and flavor it with a little honey.

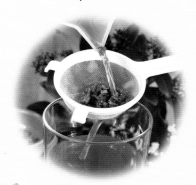

Tinctures

With a tincture, the active element of a herb is extracted using alcohol—usually vodka or grain alcohol because they have less taste than other spirits. The resulting rich liquid provides an easy-to-take solution which can either be added to water and drunk, or one or two drops placed under the tongue. It is far easier to buy tinctures ready-made but if you do wish to make your own try using echinacea or root ginger.

One of the reasons tinctures are so popular with herbalists is because they enable the body to absorb the properties of a healing herb almost immediately.

Tinctures begin to be absorbed as soon as they are in your mouth and the alcohol ensures that they are absorbed more rapidly into your bloodstream. If you don't want to use alcohol, heat the tincture first or put it in hot water so the alcohol evaporates.

You will need

• 1 oz dried or 2 oz fresh herb

• 9 fl oz brandy or vodka

• 5 fl oz water

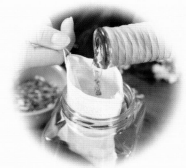

Method

1. Cut your herbs into small pieces or crush them with a rolling pin.

2. In a jar with a tight-fitting lid, mix the alcohol and water together. Add the herbs and ensure they are well covered.

3. Close the jar and store in a cool, dark place for 2-4 weeks and remember to shake the mixture every day.

4. Strain the mixture through a coffee filter, fine cloth, or muslin bag and collect the tincture liquid in another container below.

5. Store the tincture in clean, dark glass containers or store away from sunlight. If stored correctly it will last for a year.

Potpourri and Herb Pillows

Potpourri was traditionally used to mask bad smells and keep households fragrant, whereas herb pillows are a traditional remedy for headaches. Ironically the French term potpourri originally meant rotten pot. It was made with salt and fresh or semi-dried flowers to create a strong, long-lasting scent.

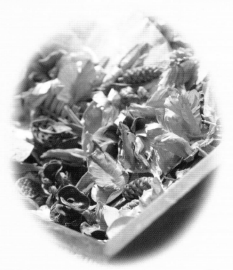

Potpourri Ingredients

You can create your own potpourri using any mix of herbs, flowers, spices, and essential oils, and you can vary the amounts until you are happy with your scent. The herbs you use could include mint, lemon balm, bay, or basil. Rosemary, thyme, and lavender become more fragrant when dried.

Sweet-scented rose petals are most commonly used but you could try lavender, violets, or carnations. Adding spices such as cinnamon, or woods such as sandalwood or cedar, and dried orange or lemon peel will also greatly enhance the fragrance. The essential oil you use could be lavender, orange, or rose. Your local health food store or pharmacy will stock all you need.

Creating Potpourri

1. Dry your flowers and leaves until they're crisp (see page 9 and follow drying herbs).

2. Place the dried flowers and leaves in a container—don't use plastic as it will absorb the aroma.

3. Add your spices, herbs, aromatic woods and citrus peel and a little powdered orrisroot to fix the aroma. Mix gently, but thoroughly, with your hands—it's a good idea to wear rubber gloves as the scent is powerful and will stay on your hands.

4. Add an essential oil of your choice (it's best to match them with your mix so lavender oil if you've used dried lavender) one drop at a time and mix again.

5. Place the mixture in large jars or freezer bags and make sure they're sealed tightly. Leave the mixture for six weeks so that it matures properly and remember to shake them every day.

Herb or Dream Pillow

These were traditionally used to treat headaches or simply to relax the sleeper.

You will need

• 2 cotton pillowcases; one will form the outer decorative cover, the other will hold the herbs and stuffing

• Dried herbs and flowers—try an equal mix of rose petals, chamomile and lavender

• Essential oil—for example lavender, jasmine, or rose

• Orrisroot powder, to fix the scent. (You may have to search for this, but if you have access to the internet, small amounts, perfect for your pillow, can be bought)

• Pillow stuffing

• Velcro, the length of the pillow opening

Method

1. Attach the velcro to the end of your inner pillowcase.

2. Fill the inner pillowcase with the herbal mixture, oil, and orrisroot until you're happy with the fragrance. Add the stuffing and close the opening, stitching if necessary. Cover with the second pillowcase.

Compresses and Poultices

Compresses and poultices are some of the oldest forms of herbal remedies. They're also very easy to make.

Compresses

Anyone who's used a washcloth to ease a fever will have experienced the benefits of a compress in its simplest form. In terms of herbal remedies a compress is a soft cloth soaked in a hot or cold infusion (pages 10-11) or decoction (page 12). A cold compress can help ease a fever or inflammation, or help tone and stimulate the body. A hot compress helps to relax and ease discomfort from cramps, aches, and pains. Before using any compress, hot or cold, perform a patch test to check for skin sensitivity (see page 6).

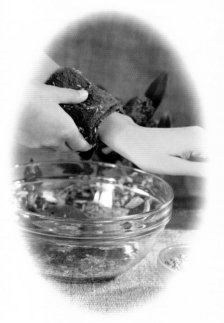

When applying a compress, squeeze out any excess water and, if using a hot compress, you can also apply a vegetable oil to the affected area to avoid scalding the skin. Also, try placing a hot-water bottle or ice pack on top of the compress to stop the temperature from changing too quickly. See pages 33, 43, and 44 for remedy suggestions.

Poultices

Poultices can be applied hot or at room temperature. Freshly crushed herbs can be used but poultices are a great use for the leftover pulp from your infusions or decoctions, especially if used while still hot from the brewing (allow some time for the pulp to cool though, it shouldn't be much hotter than body temperature). Poultices can help improve circulation, relieve spasms, tension, and pain, reduce infections and inflammation and draw out the toxins to help heal bruising, swelling, and minor wounds (leave the treatment of open wounds to a trained doctor). See pages 29, 33, and 37 for suggested poultices.

You can leave a poultice on a person overnight but not for more than ten hours at a time and it can only be used once. Don't forget to do a patch test before trying the poultice.

You will need

• Damp herb material, strained from an infusion or decoction, squeeze to remove excess water

• 1 tbsp vegetable oil (optional)

• Use fresh herbs, chopped or crushed finely, as an alternative to the damp herb material

• Thin gauze such as stretched muslin

• Cloth or plastic wrap

• Surgical tape (available from a drug store)

Method

1. Place the herbs either directly on to the affected skin or wrap the pulp in thin gauze first. If the pulp is still hot, rub a little vegetable oil onto the skin before applying the poultice to protect the skin.

2. Use the plastic wrap or cloth to keep the poultice in place, using the tape to secure it as necessary.

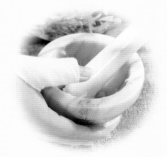

Syrups and Salves

Syrups and salves take more preparation than the remedies previously featured, but they can be made ahead of time and stored in either the refrigerator or in a cool, dark place. They make a great addition to the family's first-aid kit.

Syrups

As you would expect, syrups are ideal for easing the discomfort of sore throats and coughs. Take as directed below at the first sign of discomfort.

You will need

- 1 oz fresh or ½ oz dried herbs
- 9 fl oz boiling water
- 4 ½ fl oz honey (any honey will do)
- 1 tsp brandy or vodka (optional)

Method

1. In a saucepan, cover the herbs with the water and simmer for 20-30 minutes as you would for a decoction.

2. Stain off the herbs but return the liquid to the saucepan and simmer until the volume has halved.

3. Add the honey and heat until the honey has completely dissolved. At this point you can add the alcohol if using; it will help prevent the mixture from splitting once cooled.

4. Leave to cool slightly before transferring to dark, glass bottles and store in the refrigerator. The syrup can be taken 3-5 times a day, either a teaspoon at a time, or dissolve two teaspoons in warm water and drink like a tea. See page 43 for a good cough syrup suggestion. You can keep the syrup in your refrigerator for up to a week.

Words of Caution

Don't give unpasteurized honey to children under two.

Salves

Salves or ointments are made using infused oils and beeswax; they are only ever used externally, but you should always do a skin patch test before applying salve from a new batch or recipe (see page 6).

The greasy nature of salves provides a protective and healing barrier making them particularly good at treating rough and dry skin. Applied as part of a massage they are also good for easing muscular pain. See pages 33, 44, and 45 for suggestions and pages 23 for an anchusa lip balm.

You will need

• 2 fl oz (4 tbsp) infused oil (either your own homemade oil, see page 11, or you can buy it ready-made from your local herbal remedy or good food store)

• ½ oz (1 tbsp) grated beeswax (available in pure form from most hardware stores)

Method

1. Over a saucepan of boiling water, place the oil in a glass bowl and heat gently.

2. Melt the beeswax into the oil, stirring constantly until the wax has dissolved.

3. Remove from the heat and allow the salve to cool slightly before transferring to a shallow jar or pot. Allow to completely cool

in the container and store in a cool place out of direct sunlight. Apply as needed. Varying the amount of beeswax will affect the viscosity of the salve.

Note

Infused oils are not the same as essential oils, which are more concentrated. If you are using essential oils, dilute one drop in every tablespoon of carrier oil, such as sunflower or olive oil.

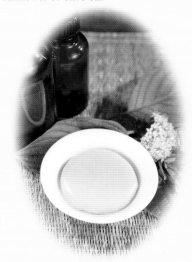

Agrimony

The name agrimony is from the ancient Greek *Argemone,* a name reputedly given to plants with healing qualities for the eyes.

Agrimony, also known as Church Steeples, grows abundantly in the countryside especially on the sides of fields, hedges, and on waste ground. It is well-known as a popular medicinal herb.

A member of the rose family, agrimony blooms from June to early September. The whole plant is deep green with leaves that vary in size. It usually grows to around 24 inches. Its flowers are small and have five egg-shaped petals.

The flowers of the agrimony plant are particularly beautiful and make it one of the most attractive herbs found growing wild. It is also a pleasantly aromatic plant.

Common Agrimony
(*Agrimonia eupatoria*)

Healing Properties

Throughout history, agrimony has been widely regarded as a powerful healing herb. The Anglo-Saxons called it *garclive* and used it for healing wounds, snakebites, and warts. One eccentric writer even recommended that it be taken with a mixture of pounded frogs and human blood as a remedy for internal hemorrhages!

In the Middle Ages, it was said to have magic powers. The great 17th century herbalist, Nicholas Culpeper, praised agrimony, saying that a decoction of the herb "is good against the biting and stinging of serpents… it also helpeth the colic, cleanseth the breath and relieves the cough".

In Culpeper's time agrimony had a great reputation for curing jaundice and other complaints and was considered a useful agent in skin eruptions and diseases of the blood and pimples. A strong decoction of the root and leaves sweetened with honey or sugar, was used to cure scrofulous sores. It needed to be taken three times a day in wineglass doses for several months, which required a great amount of dedication for the cure to work.

While the English enjoyed an infusion of the dried leaves in what was called a "spring drink" which was taken as a measure to purify the blood, the French drank infusions of agrimony as much for its fragrance as anything else. Herbalists today use agrimony to help treat coughs, sore throats, diarrhea, and indigestion.

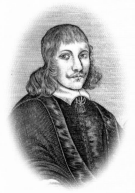

Nicholas Culpeper

Herbal Remedy—Decoction

You will need

- 1½-2 oz agrimony stem, fresh or dried
- 2 pints boiling water

Method

1. Make your decoction in the normal way (see page 12).

2. Allow the mixture to cool completely and then use the decoction as a gargle for a cold.

3. Alternatively, make an infusion with the leaves or flowers and drink a cup of the cold tea three or four times a day to ease upset stomachs.

Words of Caution

Do not use this if you are pregnant and avoid use if suffering from constipation.

Anchusa

Anchusa is a biennial herb that flowers between late May and October, it is used as a detoxing diuretic and to soften and protect the skin.

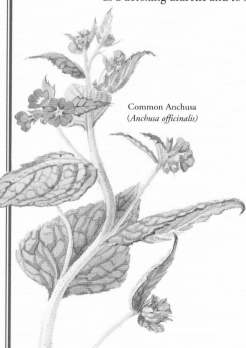

Common Anchusa
(*Anchusa officinalis*)

The charm of a flowering anchusa, also known as alkanet and common bugloss, ensures its place in many a country and urban garden. Anchusa grows to between 11-35 in. tall. It has delicate purplish blue flowers that are tubular and about an inch across with tiny, nut-like fruit. It is also excellent for attracting bees and other insects.

Healing Properties

Traditionally, anchusa was used to treat persistent coughs. In his *New Family Herbal*, published in England in 1810, Dr Robert Thornton also noted anchusa's healing properties with regard to "the cure of melancholia and other hypochondrial diseases", when steeped in strong ale and wine. Modern herbalists use an infusion of anchusa leaves and root to create remedies to break down and help dispel phlegm and mucus in the respiratory passages. It is also widely added to skin-softening remedies.

Herbal Remedy—Lip Salve

Anchusa root, normally sold in powdered form, adds a rich red color to natural lip salve as well as helping to protect and soften lips. You can experiment with the amount of anchusa root you use when deciding on the lip balm color.

You will need

• A small pinch of powdered anchusa root (this can be hard to come by so start searching well in advance before attempting this remedy. You may have to order from your nearest herbal remedy store otherwise you will have to order directly from the internet)

• 4 fl oz (8 tbsp) almond carrier oil or grapeseed oil (available from your local herbal remedy store, good food store or from the internet)

• 1 oz (2 tbsp) beeswax, grated

• 2 tsp honey

• Rose essential oil (optional, but add no more than 6 drops. Always read the manufacturer's precautions first)

Method

1. In a bowl resting over gently simmering water (a bain-marie), heat the anchusa in the carrier oil for about 15-20 minutes.

2. Strain the liquid through either a double layer of cheesecloth, a muslin bag, or a fine-meshed strainer.

3. Add the beeswax, honey, and essential oil. Heat until the honey and wax are totally dissolved and remove from the heat.

4. Test for consistency by placing a tablespoon of the oil in your freezer for five minutes. If the batch is too hard add a little more almond oil to soften it—should it be too soft, add more beeswax. Return the mixture to the bain-marie to heat until any additions have dissolved again.

5. Pour the mixture into small containers and leave to set. There should be enough salve to fill several small containers. Before use, test the salve with a patch test (page 6) and if safe apply lightly to the outer surfaces of your lips when necessary.

Words of Caution

Not to be taken while pregnant.

Elder

Elder has been described as the medicine chest of country folk, for every possible part of the tree—bark, leaves, flowers, berries—can be used in healing remedies.

Elder
(*Sambucus nigra*)

With its masses of creamy-white, fragrant blossoms, followed by the large, drooping bunches of purplish-black juicy berries, the elder is a very familiar sight in the countryside and in many North American gardens. It is said that the summer hasn't really arrived until the elder is fully in flower (mid-June) and that it is only really over when the berries are ripe.

Folklore and superstitions are richly associated with the elder and in ancient times the tree was believed to protect from disease and evil and bring good luck—reason enough for an elder tree to be planted outside England's royal cathedral, Westminster Abbey. It is also said that if you chance to fall asleep under an elder tree you'll have visions of fairyland.

Healing Properties

The bark, leaves, flowers, and berries of the elder are used in many herbal remedies. The leaves and bark of elder trees possess cleansing qualities and are useful diuretics.

Green elder ointment uses the leaves of the tree and various fats to create a remedy for the treatment of bruises and chilblains. It's also applied to wounds and used to soften and protect the skin.

Elderflowers are used to make elderflower water. This was traditionally used in mixing medicines, particularly eye and skin lotions as it's both a mild astringent as well as a weak stimulant. Edwardian ladies also swore by elderflower water to keep the complexion free from freckles, sunburn, and other blemishes.

Elderflower tea was regarded as a splendid spring medicine and, taken every morning before breakfast, as a most excellent purifier of the blood. Cold elderflower tea was used to reduce inflammation around the eyes.

Elderflower tea is recommended to treat coughs, sore throats, allergic rhinitis, and hay fever. Elderberry extract is also good for colds, flu, and irritated intestines and is available in most good food stores.

Herbal Remedy – Infusion

You will need

- 2 tsp dried elderflower
- 9 fl oz boiling water
- 1 tsp honey (optional)
- 1 tsp lemon juice (optional)

Method

1. Dried elderflowers should be available from any herbal remedy or good food store.

2. Place two teaspoons of the crumbled, dried elderflowers into a cup and pour boiling water over them. Leave to steep for a few minutes then strain and enjoy. Should you prefer, you can sweeten your infusion with honey and add a dash of fresh lemon juice to liven up the taste.

Words of Caution

Use a low concentration before trying the infusion properly.

Feverfew

Feverfew—the name relates to the herb's fever-reducing properties—grows wild in the hedgerows and has long been a favorite of country herbalists.

A perennial, feverfew has many small, daisy-like heads of yellow flowers with white outer petals. It is a pungent herb, having a bitter smell that bees, in particular, dislike.

If you wish to grow your own feverfew, the best time to plant is around the end of April. Your soil needs to be well-drained and enriched with manure. Once you've planted feverfew, it needs little attention, growing to about 24 inches.

Feverfew
(*Chrysanthemum parthenium*)

Healing properties

As well as lowering fevers, feverfew has traditionally been used in an infusion to treat hysterical complaints, nervousness, and has even been used as a tonic. Evidence suggests that at one time it was a popular cure for earache.

Bruised and heated, or fried with wine and oil, feverfew was applied externally to relieve wind and colic. A tincture made from feverfew was also said to repel insects and vermin.

As a decoction feverfew helps with coughs, wheezing, and breathing difficulties. One of the more mysterious claims made for feverfew surrounds its purifying qualities—it is said that placing it around your house will ward off disease.

Today, feverfew is mostly used to ease migraines, irregular or painful periods, joint inflammation and pain, and to reduce fevers. Typically, the fresh herb can be eaten directly, a couple of leaves at a time, or made into a tea. Tablets and prepared tinctures are also readily available.

Herbal Remedy—Infusion

An infusion of fresh feverfew leaves is the easiest ways to gain the benefits of this herb. Follow the directions on pages 10-11 but allow to cool before drinking.

Words of Caution

Do not take while pregnant, or if taking warfarin or any other blood-thinning medication. Eating the fresh leaves can cause mouth ulcers in some people.

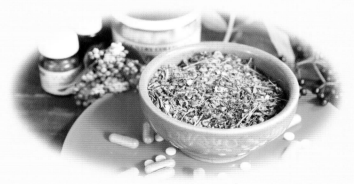

Garlic and Wild Garlic

Garlic and wild garlic has a number of uses and is a true wonder of the natural world. With its antibacterial, antiviral, antifungal, and antiparasitic properties it can be used in a number of ways to heal the body.

Garlic gets its name from the Anglo-Saxon for spear (gar) and plant (lic) and refers to the shape of its leaves.

Wild garlic or ransom is found growing wild in the countryside and is most easily discovered by following your nose. Wild garlic flowers are found at the end of a stalk that rises directly from the bulb and are white. Garlic flourishes in moist, sandy soil. If you want to grow your own simply break a garlic bulb into cloves and plant directly into the ground.

Your garlic beds need to be in a sunny spot and kept free from weeds. If you plant early in February or March, the bulbs will be ready by August. If you plant near your roses you will get the added benefit of keeping black fly away.

Wild Garlic
(*Allium ursinum*)

Healing Properties

The benefits of garlic can be accessed in a number of ways as the cloves can be eaten raw or cooked with food, rubbed on to the skin or, today, you can also choose from one of the many tablets and capsules available.

The use of garlic as a healing herb is not a recent practice; ancient Egyptian manuscripts recommended garlic for headaches, throat disorders, and physical weakness. As recently as World War I garlic was used as an antiseptic to treat infected wounds. At one time, garlic was believed to help treat both leprosy and smallpox.

Medical research continues into the benefits of garlic and many people take garlic daily to help keep their circulation healthy and to thin their blood. It has been proven to help lower blood pressure and cholesterol counts. Garlic helps with the treatment of flu, skin problems and digestive infections.

Herbal Remedy—Poultice

While simply rubbing the cut side of a clove on a spot can help treat it, a poultice of garlic can make a good treatment for viral skin infections such as warts.

You will need

• A clove of garlic

• Vitamin E oil: a few drops of liquid can be extracted from capsules available from your local drug store.

• Stretched muslin bag or strip of natural cloth

• Surgical tape or bandage tape

Method

1. Using a pestle and mortar, crush the garlic into a soft pulp.

2. As the essential oils in the raw garlic can irritate the skin, protect the wart and skin with a little vitamin E oil. Apply the crushed garlic on top of the affected area.

3. Cover the poultice with the bandage and tape in place. Leave on for 24 hours then remove. A blister should form, with the wart falling off within a week.

Words of Caution

Not to be taken with anti-clotting medication. Avoid medicinal doses while pregnant or breast-feeding—taken while nursing can worsen a baby's colic.

Heartsease

Heartsease is also known as Wild Pansy, Love-Lies-Bleeding,
Meet-Me-In-The-Entry, or Stepmother.

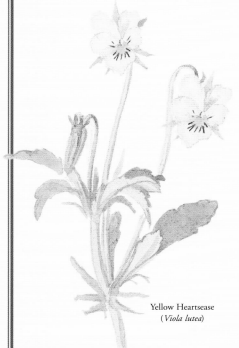

Yellow Heartsease
(*Viola lutea*)

The name Stepmother is most commonly
used in France and Germany and is an
imaginative reference to the different
shaped petals of the flowering plant. These
are supposed to represent a stepmother, her
daughters, and stepchildren.

This annual herb grows abundantly
throughout the countryside, on hedgerows
and on waste ground. Its pretty, small
flowers—either purple, yellow, white, or a
mixture—blossom from early summer
through to late autumn. To protect itself
against rain, the flower droops its head at
night and in wet weather so that the back
of the flower takes in the moisture.

Healing Properties

The heartsease plant should be harvested
between June and August when its foliage is
most abundant. The entire plant, including
seeds, should be dried in the usual way.

Over the centuries, heartsease has been used as a remedy for epilepsy, asthma, and diseases of the heart. The name may well have come about because of the belief that it was a powerful love potion.

A poultice or ointment of heartsease has been used to treat eczema and other skin complaints and is still considered an effective remedy today. Modern herbalists also use the herb to treat painful urinary conditions such as cystitis, respiratory complaints, and to reduce blood pressure.

Herbal Remedy—Infusion

You will need

- 9 fl oz boiling water
- 1 tsp dried heartsease

Method

1. Make your infusion in the normal way (page 10) and leave to infuse for 10 minutes.

2. The tea should be drunk three times a day. Alternatively make a tincture of the herb (see page 13), drink half a teaspoon three times a day.

Words of Caution

Excessive use of heartsease remedies can lead to skin problems as well as affecting cardiac function. Heartsease is also a mild laxative.

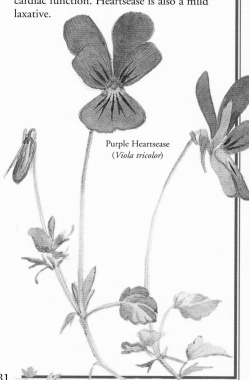

Purple Heartsease
(*Viola tricolor*)

Lavender

Lavender originally comes from the mountainous regions of those countries that border the western half of the Mediterranean—but is cultivated commercially worldwide.

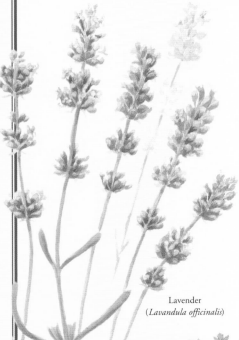

Lavender
(*Lavandula officinalis*)

For many years lavender has been valued for the fragrance of its oil. In the 19th and early part of the 20th centuries, vast areas of Europe were given over to its commercial cultivation and it is now one of the most popular herbs in the country. But, although the plant is aromatic, the oil is only produced from the flowers and flower stalks. Dried lavender is also used for fragrance, particularly in potpourri.

English lavender, the most common and most fragrant variety, grows between 12-35 inches. It has a short, irregular stem with branches covered in a yellowish-gray, thin bark. Lavender prefers to grow on light, dry soil, in an open and sunny spot. You'll need to make sure the soil is drained and free from damp in winter. Harvesting lavender is a rather complicated process but you will be able to dry the flowers. These will contain around 1.5-3 percent oil.

Healing Properties

The essential oil of lavender is an effective means to combat stress, insomnia, and headaches as the oil is known for its calmative properties. A few drops massaged into the temples or dropped onto a pillow can ease symptoms.

Lavender is anti-inflammatory and antimicrobial making the essential oil a potent remedy for irritations of the skin—including insect bites, stings, and rashes. The essential oil can also promote healing and disinfect wounds, while a lavender salve (see page 19) if massaged into muscle aches can bring some pain relief. During a fever, a tepid compress (page 16) with a few drops of the essential oil can be cooling.

Herbal Remedy—Poultice

This remedy is more of a hand mask than a traditional poultice but it does need to stay on the hands for 15 minutes in which time the honey and oil will moisturize the hands while the lavender will soothe the skin.

You will need

• 1 tsp almond or vegetable oil (available from your drug store or supermarket)

• 1 tsp honey

• 2 drops essential lavender oil

Method

1. Mix all the ingredients together then rub on to freshly washed, slightly damp hands.

2. Leave on the skin for 15 minutes then rinse off with warm water.

Words of Caution

Avoid large quantities during pregnancy.

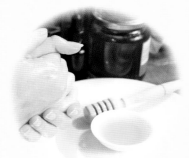

Meadowsweet

Meadowsweet is a well-known and popular British wildflower and was one
of three herbs held most sacred by the ancient druids.

Meadowsweet or
Queen of the Meadow
(*Spiraea ulmaria*)

The plant flowers from June to September
and is recognizable by its fern-like foliage
and delicate creamy-white flowers. These
are small, clustered close together and have
a pleasant, pungent smell. Meadowsweet
leaves are also very fragrant but in a
different way from the flowers. Their smell
is like almonds and in centuries past they
were strewn on the floors of banqueting
halls to make the "heart merrie and joyful"
and to delight the senses.

The herb was also known as the mead or
honey-wine herb and its dried flowers were
often put into wine and beer. You might
like to try this yourself. A handful of the
flowers will do, but let it marinate for a
while before drinking.

Healing Properties

You only use the flowers and flowering tops
of meadowsweet, fresh or dried.

Modern herbalists use the herb much in same way it always has been used: to treat the common cold, flu, general joint pain and inflammation, osteoarthritis, and rheumatoid arthritis.

Meadowsweet contains salicylic acid—the base component of aspirin—which makes it useful as an anti-inflammatory and in bringing down fever.

Unfortunately, you would need to take around 2-3 ounces of meadowsweet a day to achieve an aspirin-like effect—which is not advised! But, although the herb is nowhere near as powerful as aspirin, you should still not take it if you are allergic to the drug.

The usual amount that herbalists recommend you take is around one teaspoon of the flower a day for minor aches and pains, and mild fevers. In tincture form, take one and a half teaspoons a day.

Herbal Remedy—Infusion

Try making a decoction or infusion of the herb in the usual way (see pages 10-13).

Words of Caution

Not to be taken while pregnant or breast-feeding, or by anyone with a blood-clotting disease or those taking anticoagulants. Meadowsweet must never be given to children to reduce fevers.

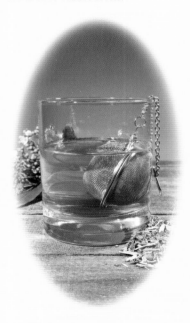

Mint

There are many different members of the mint family, including common garden mint, spearmint, peppermint, pennyroyal, and bergamot mint.

Peppermint
(*Mentha piperita*)

Mint originated in Europe and Asia but has naturalized well throughout North America. The herb is used widely in cooking, particularly with lamb or peas, but is also a common ingredient in herbal remedies.

It is a perennial herb with erect, square stems that rise to about 24 in. and bear short-stalked, pointed, and wrinkled bright green leaves. The surface of the leaf is smooth and the underneath ribbed. The plant's flowers are small and densely arranged, usually pinkish or lilac-colored.

If you want to grow your own mint, plant in the coolest and dampest part of your garden, avoiding dry, sandy soil. Mint should be harvested when the plants are beginning to bloom. You should cut the stalks above the root on a dry day, after the dew has gone and before the hot sun has dried the oil out of the leaves.

Healing properties

Of the mint family, peppermint is the most frequently used in herbal remedies, particularly the essential oil.

Any member of the mint species has its uses in the treatment of indigestion, heartburn, cramps, nausea, colic, anxiety, and stress. The simplest way to enjoy the benefits of mint, whatever the variety, is in a herbal infusion (see page 10-11).

Herbal Remedy—Poultice

A plant rash, such as a nettle sting, can be soothed with a peppermint poultice that can be reapplied as often as required. The clay will help dry the irritation, while the aloe heals and the peppermint oil relieves the itching.

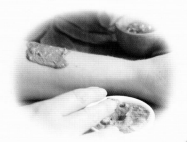

You will need

• 2 tbsp cosmetic clay or a pure clay face mask

• Aloe vera gel (to mix) available from good food stores or over the internet

• 2 drops peppermint essential oil

Method

1. Mix the clay with enough aloe vera to make a thin, smooth paste.

2. Add the peppermint oil and mix well so that it is completely combined.

3. Spread the poultice over the affected area and allow it to dry—there's no need to cover with a bandage as with other poultices. Leave on for ten minutes and wash off with warm water.

Words of Caution

Large doses of peppermint may cause epileptic seizures. Not suitable for children under 12 or while pregnant or breast-feeding. Peppermint essential oil should only be used externally and diluted with a carrier oil unless directed otherwise by a professional.

Nettle

There are as many as 500 different species of nettle worldwide, mainly tropical, although many grow in the temperate climes of Europe and Northern America.

Stinging Nettle
(*Urtica dioica*)

Although you must already know what it is like to be stung by a stinging nettle, be thankful you haven't experienced the sting of a species that grows in India. If you come into contact with this nettle the stinging sensation, caused by a liquid inside the hairs, can be agonising for hours or even days. In serious cases, the effects of being stung by the nettle can be like those of lockjaw.

The common nettle, of which herbalists use the plant and seeds, is found all over the world and is identified by its heart-shaped leaves that taper to a thin point.

Collect the whole herb in May and June, just before it comes into flower, on a fine morning when the sun has dried off the dew. Cut off the herb just above the root and tie in bunches, about 6-10 in a bunch. Obviously, you should wear gloves.

Healing Properties

The nettle's leaves are highly nutritious and when they are boiled, the young nettle leaves lose their sting and can be added to soups and casseroles.

In the past, herbalists used nettle juice to stop internal bleeding and nosebleeds. Diluted nettle juice was also used as an astringent gargle to help cure a sore throat, and nettle beer made a tasty cure for gout and rheumatism. A remedy for chronic rheumatism and loss of muscular power was to be flogged with nettles!

Modern usage of nettle utilizes the herb's diuretic, cleansing, and detoxifying properties. Nettle ointments can improve skin problems such as acne and eczema. Its astringency can help diarrhea and urinary infections as well as infections of the mouth and throat.

Herbal Remedy—Decoction

Rinse an irritated scalp with this decoction with added vinegar, combining dried nettle, rosemary, and comfrey to heal and stimulate hair growth.

You will need

- 1 tbsp dried nettle
- 1 tbsp dried rosemary
- 1 tbsp dried comfrey (omit for a rinse for dry, flaky scalps)
- 9 fl oz water
- 1 tbsp apple cider vinegar

Method

1. Mash the herbs—especially the nettle— with a pestle and mortar. Place the herbs into a saucepan with the water and bring to boil as you would for a normal decoction.

2. Once boiling remove from the heat and leave to infuse for about an hour.

3. Strain off the herb pulp, retaining the liquid. Add the vinegar to the liquid. Use at least half if not more of the mixture to rinse your scalp after shampooing. The decoction will keep in the refrigerator for two weeks.

Words of Caution

Nettle can cause some allergic reactions. Do not use while pregnant or breast-feeding.

St John's Wort

In recent years St John's wort has become popular as a natural cure for depression, even though it has been used to treat depression for centuries. Today, more than ever, it is recognized as a cure for mild depression even though scientists have no real idea how the herb works.

Small Upright St John's wort
(*Hypericum perforatum*)

Trailing St John's wort
(*Hypericum humifusum*)

St John's wort is a tough plant that grows between 12-36 in. tall. It is covered with charming, fragrant yellow flowers from mid to late summer. You should harvest the flowers when they are fully open and only pick the quantity of leaves you need.

The herb can be found growing wild but if you want to grow your own, it does best planted in average soil in dappled shade or full sun. The plants grow rapidly but are short-lived.

Healing Properties

The dried leaves and flowers of St John's wort have been traditionally used to treat a number of mental disorders and as a sedative, a balm for wounds, burns, insect bites, and even as a treatment for malaria.

Today, apart from as a treatment for depression, St John's wort is taken to moderate anxiety or sleep disorders. It is also regarded as a liver tonic and booster.

The herb is usually available in capsules and normally needs to be taken for several weeks for a noticeable effect to be seen.

Herbal Remedy—Infused Oil

An interesting remedy you might like to try uses a cold infused oil of St John's wort to relieve muscle ache.

You will need

• a handful of St John's wort flowers

• olive oil (to cover, approx. 5-7 fl oz)

• muslin (cut a muslin bag if you can't get hold of it in single sheets)

Method

1. Begin by harvesting the flowers when they are only just open. Leave them to wilt overnight, to rid them of any excess moisture that could cause the oil to mould.

2. Chop up the flower heads, put them in a glass jar and cover with the olive oil to about a depth of two inches. Cover the jar with several layers of clean muslin and secure with a rubber band—don't use a tight fitting lid.

3. After three weeks, strain the oil through fresh muslin and rebottle in a dark glass container. Store in a cool, dark place.

4. Massaging the oil directly onto sore muscles will ease the ache. Remember to perform a patch test first (page 6).

Words of Caution

St John's wort can cause sensitivity to light, so avoid long exposure to sunlight or discontinue use. If you are taking any medication at all, including the contraceptive pill, consult your doctor before use of any remedy containing this herb. Do not use during pregnancy and while breast-feeding and avoid taking with foods that contain tyramine, for example cheese and red wine.

Thyme

The most commonly found species of thyme, garden thyme, is cultivated originally from the mountains of Spain and other countries bordering the Mediterranean.

Thyme
(*Thymus vulgaris*)

The name thyme was first given to the plant by the Greeks and referred to its sweet smell. It was being cultivated across Europe by the middle of the 16th century. Garden thyme has a pleasant aromatic smell, due to an oil found in the leaves. This is used for both culinary and medicinal purposes. The plant flowers from May to August.

If you wish to grow garden thyme yourself, sow in the middle of March or early April in dry, mild weather. Thyme thrives when it has lots of room in which to spread out.

Wild thyme is found mainly on heaths, in valleys, and along ditches. Its presence supposedly indicates a pure atmosphere. There are also other varieties of thyme, including thyme basil and the wonderfully fragrant lemon thyme, which you might also wish to grow in your herb garden.

Healing Properties

Fresh or dried, the whole herb is used and its essential oil is also distilled. It can be used as an antiseptic, antispasmodic, and calmative. Wild thyme, in particular, is thought to be a good remedy for chest and respiratory infections and digestive complaints.

Culpeper recommended an infusion of thyme for treating whooping cough, nightmares and curing drunkenness. Modern herbalists have found that hot thyme infusions will induce sweating— making them useful for reducing fevers.

Taken long term, thyme helps boost the nervous system and enhances immunity. It can therefore help with mental and physical exhaustion.

Antimicrobial and astringent properties make thyme compresses useful for treating athlete's foot and other skin irritations.

Herbal Remedy—Syrup

A thyme syrup will help relax and soothe the respiratory tract to provide relief from nagging coughs.

You will need

- 9 fl oz boiling water
- 1 oz (2 tbsp) dried thyme
- 4 ½ fl oz honey

Method

1. Prepare the syrup as stated on page 18, adding the alcohol as well if you intend the syrup to last a little bit longer than a couple of days.

2. Take teaspoonfuls of the mixture as required. For an alternative syrup, halve the quantity of thyme but add tablespoons of dried liquorice and aniseed.

Words of Caution

Avoid use while pregnant or breast-feeding. Use with care if suffering with a thyroid condition as excessive use can cause overstimulation of the thyroid gland. If you experience diarrhea or bloating, cut back on the amount or discontinue use.

More Healing Herbs

The ways in which herbs can be used to help heal the body are splendidly diverse and at times miraculous. Here are some more herbs and remedies you might like to try.

Arnica

Arnica is commonly used to help heal bruises and swelling. Readily available in creams and gels from main street stores, when gently rubbed on to unbroken skin it stimulates the circulation, relieving pain, and easing swelling.

Marigold

If you go to a good food store and some drug stores you'll see that marigold is available in gels, creams, and salves and is a great treatment for burns, cuts, scrapes, and insect bites. An infusion of dried marigold flowers can be made at home and used as a compress for treating impetigo blisters. Mixing cider vinegar into the infusion will create a good soak to treat athlete's foot.

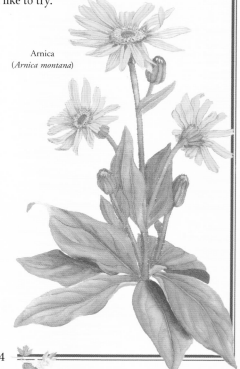

Arnica
(*Arnica montana*)

Chamomile

The dried flowers of chamomile are well-known for their relaxing properties and are commonly used in stress-relieving remedies and to aid upset stomachs.

Chamomile tea is an excellent stress-buster and can be taken at any time of day but it is best last thing at night. To aid sleep there are plenty of ready-made blends that can be bought off the shelves, but nothing quite matches a home brew infusion.

If you're using dried chamomile allow ½ fl oz of dried herb for each cup (9 fl oz) of water. Steep the herbs for ten minutes in water that has just been boiled and strain. With fresh chamomile use three teaspoons of the fresh plants to each pint of water and make in the same way.

Comfrey

Comfrey, is rich in allantoin which helps refresh, regenerate, and nourish the skin by speeding up growth in the skin cells. After a cut has scabbed or a blister burst try applying a comfrey salve to quicken the healing process. Never apply to an open wound as it can lead to the growth of abscesses.

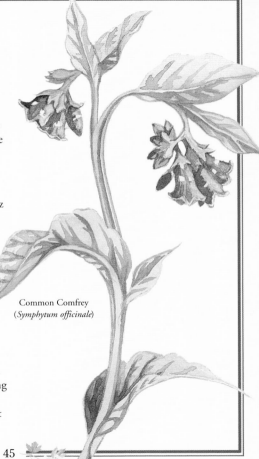

Common Comfrey
(*Symphytum officinale*)

Echinacea

Although echinacea is a North American plant, herbal remedies featuring this herb adorn the shelves of supermarkets around the world. Taking echinacea will certainly lift the immune system making it good for colds and flu. If taken at the first sign of a cold, it will generally reduce the severity and length of the symptoms but it shouldn't be taken continually for more than two months. Applied externally in lotions or creams it can treat cuts, infections, and scrapes.

Ginger

There are many ways to take ginger and enjoy its medicinal properties; the root can be eaten raw, used in cooking, or used in an infusion; it can be bought in capsules, tinctures, and as an essential oil (which should only be used externally).

The warming and stimulating effects of ginger make it good at easing the discomfort of chilblains and arthritis. The diluted essential oil can be used as a massage oil to relieve muscular aches and pain. Ingested, ginger is good for nausea, indigestion, and for colds and flu, but should be avoided by those with peptic ulcers.

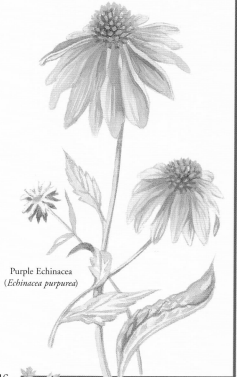

Purple Echinacea
(*Echinacea purpurea*)

Marshmallow

The squidgy sweet owes its name to this plant that grows in salt marshes. Years ago, the mucilage extracted from its roots was used to make the camp fire favorite although an artificial ingredient is used today.

As a herbal remedy, the mucilage from the root has soothing, cooling, and moisturizing properties. The root can therefore be used in infusions for sore throats (especially good if combined with ginger and peppermint) and tickly coughs as a syrup. It can also help irritation of the stomach and bowels.

Externally, a poultice of marshmallow will cool rashes and bites. To experience a herbal bath to soften dry skin, mix two tablespoons of the following: dried marshmallow root, dried comfrey leaves, dried rose petals, and dried chamomile petals. Secure the mix in a muslin bag and add to a running bath.

Rosemary

Rosemary is another herb that has been used for medicinal and culinary purposes for centuries. The herb stimulates the nerves and circulation and also helps calm the digestive system. A weak infusion of rosemary may help to relieve indigestion.

Rosemary has great antiseptic properties, making it effective in relieving sore throats. Just put three drops of rosemary essential oil into a bowl of boiled water. Hold your head about six inches from the bowl, using a towel to focus the steam towards your face. Take six deep breaths. Repeat three times in five minute intervals. If you suffer from asthma, consult a doctor before attempting this herbal remedy.

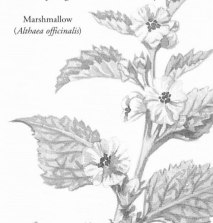

Marshmallow
(*Althaea officinalis*)

Herbs and Your Life

The reason Edith Holden's diary retains its popularity is because her own love of nature, in all its variety, is as relevant today as it ever was.

In the same way, learning about herbs allows you to understand how nature can help us, particularly at a time when life is becoming ever more complex. Most herbs can be bought easily, prepared simply, and are very good for you.

It is worth remembering that herbal remedies should be part of an everyday routine, rather than a quick fix for a possibly deeper-rooted problem.

Understanding herbs and how they work is certainly one way for you to balance the life and health of you and your family for the better. Gathering herbs or growing them in your garden will also encourage you to become more active and spend time outdoors.

Hawthorn
(*Crataegus oxyacantha*)

Of course, you've only scratched the surface. There are many other herbs for you to discover as well as plenty of other fantastic healing remedies to prepare.

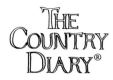

THE COUNTRY DIARY®

Other titles available in the range are:

The Country Diary of an Edwardian Lady

Herbal Remedies

Calligraphy

Flower Pressing

Cross Stitch

Learn to Paint Wildlife

Learn to Draw Nature

www.topthatpublishing.com